Cancer Advocacy For Women Simplified!

Cancer Advocacy For Women Simplified!

A WOMAN-TO-WOMAN, PHYSICIAN-TO-PATIENT CONVERSATION ABOUT CANCER

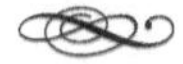

C. M. Williams, MD

ISBN: 1977751229
ISBN-13: 9781977751225

The Serenity Prayer
By Reinhold Niebuhr
God Grant me the serenity to accept the things I cannot change
The strength to change the things I can
And the wisdom to know the difference

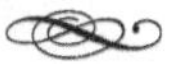

Living one day at a time,
Enjoying one moment at a time,
Accepting hardship as a pathway to peace,
Taking, as Jesus did,
This sinful world as it is,
Not as I would have it,
Trusting that You will make all things right,
If I surrender to Your will,
So that I may be reasonably happy in this life,
And supremely happy with You forever in the next.
Amen.

Contents

Foreword

We were married for thirty-eight years when we first met Dr. Williams (Doc) at Livingway Church in San Antonio, Texas. I played the saxophone in the choir, so she actually met my wife, Teresa, first. They quickly became friends as they sat in the same pew area, enjoyed praise and worship, and had that inevitable kindred and spiritual bond. Doc became good friends with our daughters as well and was considered a part of our family. We knew she had a science background but did not initially know she was an oncology physician.

I got to know Doc really well about a year later when Teresa was diagnosed with pancreatic cancer. When Doc found out what was happening to Teresa and that Teresa would need to have major surgery, known as the Whipple procedure, she was immediately in our corner, offering us support. She voluntarily met with Teresa's surgeon and her oncologist for chemo after surgery, advocating on our behalf. Doc confirmed all that was planned with the other doctors, who readily accepted her confirmations, suggestions, and knowledge. She then simplified and explained to us all the cancer medical jargon regarding what was being discussed, which helped us to understand the processes, plans, alternatives, expected side effects, and so on. It was then that I knew that Doc was sent to us by God. It was more than an eye-opening experience. It was the type of advocacy that every patient should be so fortunate to have! Before Teresa's diagnosis, we knew very little about medicine and even less of the cancer treatment process. Doc was able to comfort our family throughout Teresa's journey.

After reading *Cancer Advocacy for Women Simplified!*, I believe that this is absolutely a great and necessary work. The content is not just pages to be read, but rather it is knowledge to be learned and referred to. It is not just for the patients diagnosed with cancer but also for the caregiver of those patients. It is inspirational in that it can increase one's faith and broaden one's hope that a diagnosis of cancer should not be seen as an immediate end to life and living. This wonderful book lays out an education about cancer in an easy-to-read layman's format, encapsulating the necessary advocacy steps Doc provided for us. It provides an understanding that is vital to anyone facing such a challenge. It would be an excellent gift for loved ones, even if cancer is not present.

Teresa died in peace five years later. We were married for forty-three years. We are grateful for all the doctors and specialty staff who took care of her, the many family and friends who visited and supported us, and our Livingway Church family. But most of all, we are grateful to God for the advocate he sent us—Dr. Williams. Through this book, it is my hope that the advocacy and guidance that Doc provided to our family will be extended to you and yours.

Yours Truly,

Loren Adams,
Husband, Father, Grandfather,
Great Grandfather, Mentor, & Friend

Preface

"I AM CHOSEN. I HAVE been set apart to serve, and I do so with joy."
I did not always believe, think, or practice that phrase. But as the
years went by and I looked back at my life, I saw how the fibers of
my being were intricately weaved to achieve God's highest purpose. He has done so much with me. How can I not share? People
are perishing due to lack of knowledge, and I have been gifted to
bring wisdom and clarity. My past allows me to speak the language
of cancer such that the layman and the elite can all understand.

This book was created for my family, friends, patients and
strangers who asked my opinions about the following:

* the origin of cancer and why they got it
* the cancer-diagnosis process
* how to respond to, or handle the initial news of, cancer
  diagnosis
* how to share with others about the cancer diagnosis and
  how to handle their various responses to the news
* side effects and symptoms from treatment
* how to engage in discussions of life after cancer treatment
* intimacy and sex after treatment
* the concept of death and dying

As such, this book is a compilation of my conversations, observations, and thoughts regarding the above. This is not about one person's experience, my singular feelings, or a pure, emotional response to cancer, but a unique look at the specialty of cancer care from a physician-to-patient perspective, with transparency and compassion intertwined with God and love. This is a sister-to-sister, woman-to-woman chat about the apprehensions of the unknown throughout the cancer journey.

The Starfish Story

Original by Loren Eiseley

One day an old man was walking along the beach, when he noticed a young boy hurriedly picking up and gently throwing things into the ocean. Approaching the boy, he asked, "Young man, what are you doing?"

The boy replied, "Throwing starfish back into the ocean. The surf is up and the tide is going out. If I don't throw them back, they'll die.

The man laughed and said, "Don't you realize there are miles and miles of beach and hundreds of starfish? You can't make any difference!"

After listening politely, the boy bent down, picked up another starfish, and threw it into the surf. Then, smiling at the man, he said, "I made a difference to that one."

Life is seasonal and come in ebbs and flows. You are not alone. You do matter...

May this book be a personal guide and make a difference for you.

Peace, love, and blessings to you—*always!*

Introduction

THERE THEY WERE. MY MIND said "again," but I quickly brushed that aside. The woman was in her late sixties or early seventies, lying in a bed made up of white linen, and her arms were across her chest. She was dressed impeccably, eyes closed, still. Dead. The man in his late thirties or early forties was in the same posture and well dressed. Dead. "Where is this place?" I thought as I looked around. It was clearly not the morgue, as the usual cold, stainless-steel slabs and equipment were missing. It was not the hospital, either; the familiar beeping of vital signs by the bed, instruments hanging from the wall, monitors, and buzz at the nurses' station—none were present. It was not just quiet, it was still. A funeral home? Maybe. I could not quite see their faces, but I wondered why they would request radiation-therapy treatment for a woman who was clearly dead. I surveyed the room again. There was rustling that made my attention snap back to the beds. I gasped and looked in that direction.

"My head is hanging off the bed a bit. Help me fix it," the "dead" woman said. I hesitated, frozen. My eyes darted rapidly around to see who she was speaking to. Why was she speaking? She waited. Ever so slowly, I moved closer to the bed suspiciously. Without touching anything and being sure to keep my distance, I peered over and said, "Just wiggle down a bit." She did. My attention was startled away from her by a familiar sound to the left. The man in the other bed was now watching the television. Cartoons? Strange. I turned my attention back to the woman, but she had closed her eyes again and returned to that posture. "Hello?" I said.

She answered, "Yes."

"Why are you lying in that position? They sent me to treat you."

"I am waiting on my coffin," she said with dignity. "Be a doll and make sure my feet get in properly, would you?"

"Whaa...? But you are—not—dead." Did I say that out loud or just in my thoughts? I turned around, and it was deathly quiet again. They had both reassumed the postures and were still. Arms across their chests. No obvious signs of life. Dead. I was speechless.

Then I woke up. After a long chain of dreams that night, I was exhausted. I felt ill. My husband was already up to get our toddler son. It was Labor Day Monday and he had plans, but I was in no shape to participate. After telling him my dreams in their entirety, I ran to the bathroom. What did I watch? What did I eat? Was this a message? I think it was the latter. The message—a cancer diagnosis does not mean death. You are not dead yet. Stop pretending. Death will come in due time, but do not hasten it or waste precious time waiting. You are not dead yet!

Practicing medicine is a gift to practice art. The physician must have a certain underlying passion for what she does. Most people simply assume that all physicians have what it takes. Why else would one practice medicine? However, not everyone is strong enough to handle blood, work on a brain, fix a limb, drain the pus from a sinus, or even be around those who are ill—someone sneezes in a room and everyone covers their face and scatters from the germ bomb. When it comes to practicing oncology (cancer), it takes a special fiber that often goes unnoticed and underappreciated. The oncology team must address the shattering of people's hopes and dreams, the sudden realization that they must face death and dying, and even grimmer thoughts of long, drawn-out, painful deaths. For many patients, once diagnosed with cancer, they are like the woman in my dream—just waiting for their coffin. If you are diagnosed with cancer, understand that you are not dead yet. Until your last breath, you should live, even if it's simply because you are alive and you can still make a difference.

While attending a close family friend's funeral, I was speaking with my dad about how much she would be missed. His response was, "Well, life is a terminal disease. We all must die one day." The truth and wisdom of his statement stayed with me over the years. Cancer is not the only thing that causes people to exist in a fog, waiting on death. Life has a way of throwing curve balls of illnesses and sudden life changes. I have witnessed a variety of responses to cancer diagnoses over the years. I do not have the answers, but I hope by sharing a few things I have learned, it will set you on path of adjusted thought patterns that may help you live your life to the fullest. You are not dead *yet*; stop acting like it and start to live…again.

> *I live urgently because I walk among those who*
> *must face the concept of death and dying…*
> *constantly. Cancer is wickedly generous!*

—C. M. WILLIAMS, MD

Peace, love, and blessings to you—*always*!

CHAPTER 1

The Clouds Roll In: The Suspicion

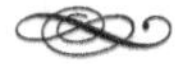

*Nothing in life is to be feared, it is only to be understood. Now
is the time to understand more, so that we may fear less.*

—MARIE CURIE

WE LIVE OUR LIVES WITH a feeling of expectancy. We anticipate
that every day will be just like the day before. We go to work, we
plan vacations, and we talk about the latest trends, news, and family celebrations; we peek at other people's life through the eyes
of social media. Living life in the fast lane is the norm for many
women who are shuffling careers and family. Multitasking is at
the core of everything we do. We have this compulsion that we
must be the best, do better, or exceed and excel in some form or
fashion. No one is exempt. The stay-at-home mom wants to make
the most creative meals, attend all the parent-teacher association
(PTA) meetings, provide great baked goods for the soccer teams,
keep a clean home, venture into entrepreneurship while watching
daytime sequels, stay beautiful (a societal moving target), and let's
not forget, pleasure herself and her mate at the end of most days.
Career women go to work early, leave late, spend hours in traffic

while doing business on the phone, strategize on how to maneuver the ladder of success, compete for positions and recognition, get or prepare dinner at home, pick up the kids, do laundry, stay beautiful (a societal moving target), and satisfy themselves and their mates at the end of most days. It's exhausting, stressful…and even sometimes depressing. Who has time for a doctor's appointment? We have much to do, and if we feel sick, we'll just check the Internet for a diagnosis, buy something over the counter, have a sugary, blended juice with a toss of vegetables, some oils, and tree leaves, and be good and ready to go in the morning. Or so we hope. It's not the correct or best approach.

Many women barely make the time for the routine annual physician visit—be it due to a lack of interest, busy schedule, no insurance, or some other form of financial hardship. Regardless of the reason, all life comes to a halt when there is an abrupt change in health, such as a cough that won't go away and/or coughing up blood, a lump in the breast or in the armpit (axilla), an ulcer/open sore on the tongue that won't heal, dark black tarry (old blood) or bright red blood on stool or toilet paper after wiping, a sore or lump in the anal area that will not go away, change in size and shape of what was thought to be a wart, fever and/or chills nightly with lumps under the arms or shoulder-blade area, persistent weakness, yellow eyes or yellow-tinged skin or stool, frequent bleeding after intercourse, bleeding years after menopause, and so on. These symptoms do not necessarily mean that you have cancer. Not all. Over 70 percent of lumps in the breast are noncancerous, bright red blood on stool or tissue could be just hemorrhoids bleeding, a persistent cough may be cold or allergy related, and intermittent fevers could be hot flashes from menopause. However, there is usually one way to know for sure, and that does *not* include your self-diagnosis. Physicians and those who know doctors are the worse culprits. Doctors tend to just ask colleagues in what we fondly call "hallway consultation" so that we can get on with our business of caring for others, forgetting about ourselves in the process. I'm guilty.

But let's be practical. What do you do when your car makes a clunky sound, it's taking a longer time than usual to start or turn over, or the engine light comes on in the dashboard? When you have a flat tire, do you keep driving it in the same condition weeks or months later? Of course not! So why do you take better care of your car than your body? Do you use premium gas in your car? You should put premium food in your body (more fruits and vegetables, for example). Do you take your car in for oil change and other routine checks? Then you should get your pap smear, mammogram, and colonoscopy—routine checks. Simple.

If you do not take care of your car, you can get another car or take public transportation (bus, train, taxi). However, if you do not take care of your body, that's it! Doctors may give you a few replacement body parts for a while, but prevention and early detection, *if possible*, are usually best.

<u>Be an Advocate</u>: *Don't know what test you should have at what age? I encourage you to speak with your Primary Care Physician (PCP) about screening for breast cancer, colon cancer, cervical cancer, and lung cancer. Ask if you are at increased risk for any particular cancer (family history of cancer, smoking history, high alcohol intake, and so on). Be sure to discuss the testing and frequency as well. If you desire to have a test done more often (for example, pap smear), let your doctor know your reasons, and arrange a more suitable frequency (every other year if normal). Insurance may or may not allow it, but you won't know if you don't ask.*

Don't be afraid to speak up and engage with your medical providers. This is your body and your temple. You only have one—take care of it.

Remember, women are the **health gatekeepers** of the family. You should know because awareness is the key. You have to know; knowledge itself is power. Now, get moving!

> *So do not fear, for I am with you; do not be dismayed,*
> *for I am your God. I will strengthen you and help you;*
> *I will uphold you with my righteous right hand.*

—Isaiah 41:10 NIV

Peace, love, and blessings to you—*always!*

CHAPTER 2

Lightning and Thunder: The Cancer Diagnosis

I know God will not give me anything I can't handle.
I just wish that He didn't trust me so much.

—MOTHER TERESA

THE UNKNOWN AND THE PROCESS of multiple tests to finding out whether cancer is present or absent can be the most anxiety-producing time in any woman's life. You might imagine the most horrendous situations of cancer progression, visible tumor growth on skin, pain and frequently think of dying an ugly death. You may even begin to think of those who have passed away from cancer or remember movies with painful endings and other scenarios that can quickly put you in a depressive mood. You are not alone. No one, and I do mean *no one*, who must travel this path will be delighted as she prepares for a mammogram, colonoscopy, or pap smear. This is a serious and somber time. The "what ifs" cloud our minds and sometimes our judgments. This is when you must dig deep and assess how you will respond, one way or another. If it is not cancer, what will you change in your life? Will you slow down? Will you eat better and exercise more? Will you quit smoking (or dipping or chewing) and decrease your alcohol intake? Get in touch with long-lost loved ones? Seek spiritual acceptance? You may say, "Doc, but I'm doing all that already—I'm a vegetarian, I exercise regularly, have no or minimal alcohol, have a relationship with God, am close to my loved ones, have no cancer in my family, don't smoke (or dip or chew), or hang with those who do—I am doing great! Cancer is not an issue for me." That is not the best mindset, as many will testify that those statements are simply not true. Many patients do all the right things and are still diagnosed with cancer. Sometimes it is due to genetics (family history), unknown exposure to chemicals that cause cancers (carcinogens such as asbestos), or random damage to cells, among other things.

The road to evaluating any abnormality is a long one. At the baseline, there will be ***radiographic imaging***, including but not limited to:

- Mammogram
- Computed Tomography (CAT/CT scan)
- Magnetic Resonance Imaging (MRI) – (If you're claustrophobic, let your doctor know. He or she can prescribe medication for relaxation.)
- Positron-Emission Tomography (PET scan)
- Ultrasound
- X-rays

Additionally, most evaluations will require a ***biopsy*** (sample of the abnormal tissue/lump) and ***bloodwork*** to evaluate whether certain organs are affected. There are many other evaluation/tests that can be done, but the above is just a start.

The worst part of the process is *waiting*. Waiting for results which may take several days, or sometimes in the case of a questionable biopsy, a couple of weeks as the doctors investigate further by seeking the advice of specialist to review the biopsy tissue samples.

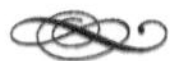

<u>Be an Advocate</u>: *When your doctor tells you that certain tests are required, be sure to ask the following:*

- *Why do I need these tests? What will the results tell us?*
- *When I complete the test/exam, how long before the results are usually available?*
- *Should I call for the results, or will you contact me?*
- *If I do not hear from you as planned, may I have information for the best way to contact you?*

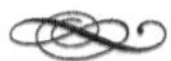

CANCER DIAGNOSIS

The "C" word is frightening to everyone. I have been blessed to serve people in all walks of life: doctors, stay-at-home moms and dads, lawyers, engineers, grocery cashiers, policewomen, firefighters, politicians, entrepreneurs, garbage collectors, school teachers...you get the picture. For all, the diagnosis is a cause for pause, a moment of somber reflection. Many patients diagnosed with cancer fear that they may have missed fulfilling their life goals and ambition, while others see it as a chance to be truthful to themselves and others and begin to make their lives more purposeful, no matter how much time is remaining. Such a diagnosis is often described as being awakened from a deep sleep by having icy water thrown in one's face. Cancer can be a comma in life for some patients, but a full stop for others. By reading this book, you are choosing a comma. You are choosing to pause only and then move on with your precious life. Know you are not alone.

There are many different cancers, and within every type of cancer, even within the same diagnosis, there are differences. "Is breast cancer the only cancer in women? " was an innocent question from a young lady in her late twenties at a general meeting. I briefly reviewed the diverse types of cancers common to women with her and encouraged her to have her first ever pap smear. We assume in the medical community that *everyone* knows how to take care of his or her body and when to get necessary screening but simply chooses not to do so. We are finding out that truthfully, many people do not know, hence the encouragement to have more in-depth and meaningful conversations with your PCP, not just to see him or her when you are ill.

When it comes to cancer diagnosis, your cancer team is interested in two broad categories to guide their treatment recommendations and discussions:

- ***Local or regional cancer***: cancer located only in the area where it started (original site, such as colon) and may include a few lymph nodes close by
- ***Metastatic cancer:*** cancer that has spread to different regions of the body (for example, from the original site of the breast to the hip bone)

There are some primary cancers that do not spread to other areas but are very serious nonetheless based on tissue biopsy and location (for example, primary brain cancer such as glioblastoma multiforme, or GBM). As noted before, there are many types of cancers, and you may get a general overview in appendix A.

Cancer Staging

Many patients are confused with the cancer-staging process. In most cases, the length of time tends to be aggravating. "Doc, I was diagnosed with cancer two weeks ago. Nothing has been done to treat it yet. They just have me doing more and more tests. What is taking so long? Isn't the cancer spreading?" a caller asked in utter frustration during a talk show. Twenty minutes later, after I skillfully questioned and attempted to calm her, she better understood the big picture. As the story unfolds, she had a visit to the Emergency Department (ED) during Thanksgiving for what was thought to be a heart attack but turned out to be acid reflux (heartburn). While in the ED, a CT scan was done to rule out a clot in the lungs (Pulmonary Embolism, PE) given her report of new onset shortness of breath. The scan did not show a clot, but it did show an enlarged lymph node in the left shoulder/front lower neck region. This led to further evaluation. The lymph node was later biopsied, but the breast estrogen and progesterone receptors were negative, and the mammogram of both breast showed suspicious calcifications with no associated mass in the right breast and nothing in the left breast (the side where the lymph node was positive for cancer). Armed with the appropriate information, I was able to provide clarification regarding her status. The area where the lymph node was biopsied (sample of tissue taken) and was positive for cancer could have originated from any of three areas in close proximity. The three areas where the cancer could have started includes:

1. The breast: doctors need to run tests on the biopsy tissue to look for breast markers. The calcifications seen on the mammogram will be compared to previous mammograms (she had not had one in the past four years) and also biopsied to look for cancer. An MRI may also be considered in some cases for further evaluation, as some breast cancer types are better seen on an MRI.

2. Head and neck cancers: cancers from the mouth and/or throat can also spread to the lower neck area, so that would involve an evaluation from the Otolaryngologist (also known as an Ear, Nose, Throat (ENT) doctors) to look for any suspicious lesions in the nose, throat and mouth.

3. Lung cancer: this cancer can also spread up to the front lower neck/shoulder area. So, the CT scan may be repeated with injected contrast material (if not used earlier) to see the organs better, and any suspicious nodules or lymph nodes in the chest (mediastinum) would also be biopsied. The team may also decide to get a PET scan to see if there is cancer anywhere else in the body.

A treatment plan cannot be made until the team knows which of the three cancers they are treating. In knowing the primary cancer location, the team can determine if it is local or regional or if it has metastasized, and they will have a better idea of their ability to control it and relay the most accurate information to the patient and family. So yes, there was still a lot of investigating to do and a few more tests to perform in this mystery. Will the cancer grow in the interim? Would the cancer be growing if acid reflux (heartburn) did not prompt an ED visit? The answer was yes to both, but the ED visit caused the cancer to be discovered much sooner than it otherwise would have been. It is a matter of perspective, but, nonetheless, an important viewpoint. Some may choose to be grateful for the acid reflux that led to the discovery of the cancer. Others might instead focus on the slow progress to getting an answer about the diagnosis and treatment recommendations and thus remain in heightened stress and possibly have a mental breakdown, thereby becoming unable to work or be there for their families. Life is a series of choices. In this case, choose calm and be grateful for the awesome Thanksgiving dinner with family and friends that caused the acid reflux. Easier said than done, but I know you can do this!

Simply put, staging is gathering all the evidence available to put a case together. What kind of cancer is it? Once that is known, the TNM staging is applied to decide on the best treatment path:

* **T (tumor)**: the size or depth of the cancer at the primary site
* **N (node)**: Are cells from the tumor starting to travel to other areas of the body? Did they get trapped by the lymph nodes? If yes, how many lymph nodes are involved? How close are the lymph nodes to the primary cancer site?
* **M (metastases)**: Did the cells from the primary cancer travel far away to new organs? Did they leave the primary site of the colon or lung and travel to the brain, liver, or bones?

Once the TNM is known, it can be further "grouped" into Stages; 0 through IV. The TNM, overall group stage, receptor status, and other special information seen under the microscope from the biopsy specimen will help your team decide on the best treatment approach. An example for breast cancer would be: **cT1cN1MX**, group **Stage IIA**. Breaking down this TNM and group Stage for better understanding is explained below:

* The small "**c**" is telling us that this staging is clinical, meaning that this staging is done prior to any treatment (for example, surgery) and is based on what was seen on the mammograms, ultrasound, and felt on the clinical exams only.

- **T1c** is telling us that the cancer size is between 1 and 2 cm (T1a would mean the cancer is between 0.1 cm and 0.5 cm; T2 would mean the cancer is between 2 and 5 cm, and so on).
- The **N1** is telling us that lymph nodes in the axilla (under the arm) are abnormal with cancer present as evident from a biopsy.
- **M0** means that there is no clinical or radiographic evidence that the cancer has spread to other areas of the body.

After the surgery, this same stage may change and would be indicated by a small "p," such as **pT1cN2M0**. The N2 would tell us that four to nine lymph nodes are positive under the arm. As you can see, this can become quite complex, but if laid out, it can be understood. Ask questions. For examples of general questions to ask to help understand the process, see appendix B and the companion book, *"Questions for Cancer Doctors - A Cancer Journal."*

Be an Advocate: *Ask your doctor to write down both your TNM stage and/or overall group stage (if it applies to your cancer). Ask if he or she can show you on an anatomic diagram, which is a drawing or picture of the body showing where the cancer is located. Knowing this information will allow you to have improved communication with other physicians and your loved ones.*

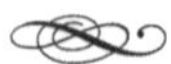

When I am afraid, I put my trust in you.

—Psalms 56:3 NIV

Peace, love, and blessings to you—*always*!

CHAPTER 3

Flood Watch: Mental Preparation for Treatment

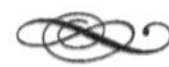

You have to accept whatever comes and the only
important thing is that you meet it with courage
and with the best that you have to give.

—ELEANOR ROOSEVELT

A GOOD FRIEND OF MINE was diagnosed with breast cancer, and I told her, "Be sure to find out if the hospital offers a multidisciplinary clinic or have a tumor board." At her next appointment, she asked the surgeon, and along with a quizzical look, his response was mumbled along the lines that they did not have a multidisciplinary clinic. She quickly interjected that her friend was an oncologist, after which the surgeon gave fire-hose answers. She was surprised at how much she understood based on our conversation combined with watching the videos on Questions4CancerDoctors.com, but the surgeon assumed she knew a lot more, too. She thought his response was "interesting" once she mentioned knowing an oncologist. (While not everyone can have a family or friend who's a physician, guides such as this one can certainly make you much more prepared.) It turns out they had a tumor board though, which is acceptable. A multidisciplinary clinic can be overwhelming, but a tumor board is usually recommended at a minimum, in some form.

A multidisciplinary clinic is quite common for breast and prostate cancer. This clinic usually involves the patient and caregivers in a single room, while other medical specialists rotate through, visiting for thirty to forty-five minutes and discussing their likely involvement in the treatment plan, expected side effects, outcomes, and so on. Another format is where the patient and caregivers sit in a conference room with all of the medical specialists while the case is presented and discussed (similar to the setting of a courtroom, with the patient being the judge, if you will, absorbing information and deciding with the team which approach of treatment they would prefer). Medical specialists include the surgical oncologist, medical oncologist, radiation oncologist, pathologist, and radiologist as the core team. Based on resources available, geneticists, physical therapists, research, nurse navigators, and behavioral health specialists (psychiatrists, psychologists, or social workers) may also be added to your team. Having a conversation with each of the above team members in one day, in either setting mentioned, can make for a long, tiring, and overwhelming day. I do not advise going to these appointments alone. Bring a family member, friend, or church member—another listening ear to help you absorb the information. If you must attend these appointments alone, then be sure to take notes using the *Questions for Cancer Doctors - A Cancer Journal* and/or ask permission to record the discussion. In some cases, I have had family members and friends call in during the discussion portion of my consultation, and with the patient's permission to discuss everything freely, they were placed on speakerphone and allowed to participate in the question-and-answer portion. Trust me, you will be grateful for the additional listening ears.

A tumor board occurs *without* the patient being present; the core medical team discusses the patient in a case format either before or after the patient has had a chance to meet with each member of the team separately. This too can be quite strenuous, as it will require juggling schedules to meet with each cancer specialist at various times, usually not all in the same week or even before a tumor board meets. If each member of the cancer team is not in the same hospital or if they do not communicate on a regular basis, then your work as an advocate is that much more intensified. You and your caregiver should try to keep track of everything. See appendix B to help you along your journey, and *"Questions for Cancer Doctors – Starter Questions to Encourage Conversations with your Cancer Team"* have general questions you may ask different specialists that you may keep as a journal of the process. Before any treatment begins, you should have the big picture and know the expected next steps or alternatives. Can you have surgery? If no, is the limitation based on your current health status (heart condition, advanced breathing condition, and so on) or the state of the cancer (for example, advanced stage, cancer wraps around or too close to vital organs)? Can you have chemotherapy alone or combined with radiation therapy to shrink the cancer and then be considered for surgery? If surgery is an option, will you have it or chemotherapy first? Do you need to have radiation therapy? Why or why not? The answers to these questions are important in establishing not only a plan, but a foundation for a positive mindset. It places you back in the driver's seat.

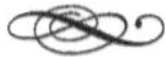

<u>Be an Advocate</u>: *If there is any hesitancy on the treatment plan on either your side or the cancer team's and you are unsure of the big picture regarding the diagnosis and treatment plan, it is perfectly OK to ask for **<u>a second opinion</u>**. A good team is never insulted by such a request, and in some cases, as physicians, we encourage and recommend a second opinion. We are confident in our recommendations, but some cases are in gray areas, and a different viewpoint can be helpful to you in the decision-making process.*

You will quickly realize that mental preparation is more than half the battle. You should be prepared to fight. Believing and standing on someone or something and knowing who is on your side will help you get ready. You cannot see, touch, or feel your thoughts, but they are there. This is spiritual warfare—do not go into battle alone.

> *Do not be anxious about anything, but in every
> situation, by prayer and petition with thanksgiving,
> present your request to God. And the peace of God,
> which transcends all understanding, will guard
> your hearts and your minds in Christ Jesus.*
>
> —*Philippians 4:6-7 NIV*

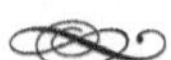

Peace, love, and blessings to you—*always*!

CHAPTER 4

Heat Wave: The Treatment Process

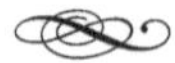

*Uncertainty is the only certainty there is, and knowing
how to live with insecurity is the only security.*

—JOHN PAULOS

NOW THAT YOU HAVE MET with all the cancer specialists and have
a better understanding of the cancer, its stage, the treatment plan,
expected side effects, possible outcomes and prognosis, and you
have a determined mindset to fight, *it is time to face off.* No two patient experiences are the same. Listening to others may help give
an overall idea of what to expect, but your outcome could be very
different. While there may be many novel and different types of
treatments, only the three most common and conventional ones
will be reviewed here. These include surgery, chemotherapy, and
radiation therapy:

- Surgery: the goal is to remove the cancer, if possible, with
  clear margins (leaving nothing behind). It is very local-
  ized, meaning if there are small cells that escape from the

18

primary tumor/cancer, the surgeons cannot see them with the naked eye and so cannot remove them. This is where chemotherapy is very helpful.

* Chemotherapy: sometimes, small cells from the cancer break away to find lodging elsewhere. Think of chemotherapy as Pac-Man who goes everywhere throughout the body, gobbling up all the cancer cells. In the process, some normal cells are also damaged. The good thing is that the normal cells can repair themselves, whereas the cancer cells, due to initial damage, do not have the ability to repair themselves and thereby are destroyed.

* Radiation therapy, which I fondly call "the healing beam" is a local treatment. Only where the beam is pointed will you be affected. If the breast is being treated, then you will not lose the hair on your head or have diarrhea because those areas are not being targeted. However, your radiation oncologist will discuss the normal tissue close by that may be affected, what to expect and measures used to decrease side effects.

While there are many theories, stories, and fabled cures for cancer, I cannot speak to any of those. Is it wise to trust a cancer treatment to unknown herbs, dietary changes, or oils? The decision is yours. No one can tell you how to keep your temple. As physicians, we are advisors who pool our data from past experiences of thousands of patients before you who entered in trials, studies, and protocols to help decide on the best treatment...*for now*. The "*now*" is a moving target, and conventional treatments and recommendations do change as new study results are made available. However, some would prefer to bet their lives on the claimed success stories of a few souls. Do not think for a moment that these herbs and oils are cheap, either. I have seen patients rack up thousands of dollars in debt for nothing short of grass and olive oil. I have a personal appreciation for alternative medicine. Once as a teenager, I stepped on a rusted nail, and Grandma scraped some mush something, added a dash of this and that and some special oil in a special prepared cloth, and bandaged it to my foot. I did not even break a fever, and in two days, I was doing just fine. Not even a limp. Would I agree with a patient that the same recipe would work for cancer? No. But many patients tend to use a similar philosophy: if something works for someone else or some other disease, then it should work for cancer. While I am always very respectful of other's work, at this point, I stick to what I know works and would not gamble anyone's life on any unknown concoction.

The spiritual questions come up in discussions, too. "Jesus will heal me. I do not need surgery, chemotherapy, or radiation therapy," some would say. Yes, Jesus does heal. He can heal miraculously, and he can heal through the hands of the surgeon, through the difficult chemotherapy, and through the healing beam of radiation therapy. Jesus healed many who were blind and afflicted, but he never healed any of the blind the same way. Faith is important, and studies have shown that those who are hopeful and have faith during treatment tend to do better overall. The story is told of a man who refused to leave his home during a hurricane because he believed God would save him. He turned away a firetruck, boat, and helicopter. He eventually drowned, and when he got to heaven, he said, "God, why didn't you save me?" God told him, "I sent a firetruck, a boat, and even a helicopter. I thought you just wanted to come home to see me." Unwavering faith is great, but do not miss that sometimes the answer may appear in a form that is not expected. Do not miss the firetruck, boat and helicopter that God may be sending your way through your oncology doctors and cancer team.

<u>Be an Advocate</u>: *The treatment process is a beast, both mentally and physically. As with anything in life, different folks will handle the process differently. Find and plug into what will make the process easier. Speak with the cancer team, support groups, mental health groups, or others who are familiar with working with patients going through treatment and/or have gone through it themselves. Be careful. Know you are unique, and as such, expect experiences to have similarities, but the differences may be greater.*

I do not have all the answers, and I'm probably not able to debate with the evangelicals of today. But what I do know is that God wants you well. Be determined to live your best life now because in the end, realize that Lazarus did die…again.

> *He gives strength to the weary and increases the power of the weak. Even youths grow tired and weary, and young men stumble and fall; but those who hope in the Lord will renew their strength. They will soar on wings like eagles; they will run and not grow weary, they will walk and not faint.*
>
> *-—Isaiah 40:29-31 NIV*

Peace, love, and blessings to you—*always*!

CHAPTER 5

Fall Foliage: Cancer Treatment Complete. Now What?

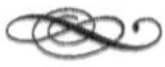

We must let go of the life we have planned, so
as to accept the one that is waiting for us.

—JOSEPH CAMPBELL

SOME PATIENTS DISLIKE THE TERM "survivor," while others embrace it. When used, an individual is considered a "cancer survivor" from the time of diagnosis through the remainder of her life. What is quite maddening to most patients is that we, as physicians, shy away from using the term "cure," but prefer instead terms such as "disease-free survival," "cancer-specific survival," and "cancer-free interval," though in radiation oncology they use the term "treatment with curative intent," which can be a source of confusion for patients. Because we can never truly mandate a "cure" or try to define it as a certain number of years from diagnosis, there exists a lingering fear of recurrence for many patients, and rightfully so. What happens when the treatments are all completed? During the treatment process, you may start with the skillful hands of a surgeon followed by the watchful eyes of the medical oncologist while chemotherapy drugs are infused and regular labs are done to assess bone marrow reserves and concerns about fevers; there are regular calls from nurses to check on your well-being. Then on to radiation therapy, if it was recommended where you are met by a great team of therapists daily and you meet and form bonds with other patients, sometimes daily for up to seven weeks. You see the radiation oncologist at least weekly and the nurse whenever you have any questions. Then treatment ends. The routines end. What now?

Once treatment is completed, a follow-up guide or a survivorship-care template should be provided to you by your cancer team. It may have a different name based on the institution, but the templates should all basically have similar content. The survivorship-care plan template outlines for you when your next follow-up appointments will be with the radiation oncologist, medical oncologist, surgeon, and any other specialist who was vital in your care. Generally, the standard for patients treated with curative intent is a follow-up plan that spans at least five years:

* every one to three months for the first two years
* every six to twelve months for the next three years

That is, you should be seen by one of your physicians at least every three months (for some cancers, such as cancers of the head and neck area, follow-up may be more frequent). The goal is not to be seen by every single physician each time, but to alternate such that someone has an eye on you every three months for the first two years and so on. Patients report that the fear sets in once the treatment is completed. The schedule change from regimented treatment to spaced-out follow-ups causes separation anxiety of sorts. Your oncology physicians and cancer team can provide the follow-up guidelines for your specific cancer. One size does not fit all, so be sure to ask.

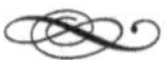

<u>Be an Advocate</u>: *Before, or at the end of your treatment for any cancer service, be sure to ask:*

* *What is the follow-up plan once my treatment is completed?*
* *Is there anything specific that should prompt me to call you or seek immediate emergency care?*
* *What are some of the late side effects that may occur?*
* *Should I expect to be (more) fatigued? Any physical limitations?*

If in pain, be sure you have a schedule for adequate pain control, or if on steroids, be sure to have written tapering-off instructions. Do not stop medications suddenly.

At a follow-up appointment, a patient said, "I have a couple more things to do, then it will back to normal. Just like it was before this cancer thing came along." I introduced the term a "new normal" and gently reminded her that striving for "how things use to be" may ultimately be very frustrating. Establishing a "new normal" was encouraged instead. The concept, though new, was well received.

If you are traversing this path, also consider a plan for psychological and spiritual support, even if you think you may not need it. Get involved in something, anything. For some, it's plugging into prayer and devotion time; for others, it's a new hobby such as knitting. Others may become active in support groups or volunteering. Whatever the choice, many survivors will tell you that this is not the time for complete isolation. Alone time for meditation to focus your mind and some introspective review is great, but time with family and friends also work wonders in the healing process. There is a time and place for everything. Balance is key.

Trust in the Lord with all your heart, and lean not on your own understanding; in all your ways acknowledge him, and he shall direct your paths.

—*Proverbs 3:5-6 NKJV*

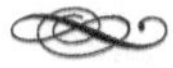

Peace, love, and blessings to you—*always!*

CHAPTER 6

Winter: Sex and Intimacy after Cancer Treatment

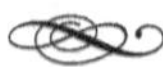

You cannot be lonely if you like the person you're alone with.

—Dr. Wayne Dyer

THE HILLS AND VALLEYS OF cancer treatment are over. You are super thankful for all the support your family, friends, and loved ones offered during this very difficult time. Now that treatment is over, your body is not the same. It will never be the same, either externally or internally. Your thoughts about life and living are not the same. For most, the appreciation of life comes into focus with quite a powerful and increased sense of awareness. Everything means more. The sun is brighter, food taste better, family and friends are more precious. Love now flows easily. Nothing is a big problem anymore, and excusing yourself from confusion and contention is easier. Then, doing a part of what we were created to do, showing physical love, presents itself. How should this be maneuvered? First, get to know you again.

GETTING TO KNOW YOU AGAIN

This, however you choose to see your position after cancer treatment, is new for you. There is a new scar on your abdomen or your chest, your breast is now missing or scarred from surgery, or your uterus was removed. New hair growth is now present, but eyebrows and lashes are still gone. Standing naked in front of a full-length mirror can be therapeutic. You must look. Touch the scars. Feel your head without hair. See yourself without makeup. Look deep into your own eyes. See you. Stand there and look. Marvel at your beauty. Be amazed at the power of your body to heal. Be impressed with your mental fortitude of getting through treatment. Smile. Try it. Just smile at the *you* that you are, the strength that you did not know was there. You are still here. Beautiful. Next, tell your significant other about the experience: what you did, how you have changed, and that you are trying to be OK with what you see in the mirror. If it was difficult for you, it will likely be slightly difficult for them as well…in the beginning. But love can see you through all things. Practice touching and looking at the area that brings the most apprehension. Know that the scars do not make you. Learn to love yourself again, and in so doing, loving your mate will follow. There is no golden time frame, seven steps, or guarantee on how the future of your relationship with your significant other will be. The most important relationship is building up yourself and standing on God's promises. Time heals all wounds, even if the scars remain. The scars are just reminders of your strength.

INTIMACY AND INTERCOURSE

Feelings of trust and intimacy must come first. To trust that your body, scars and all, will be accepted and that the touch, the care, the look, and the love are all genuine from your mate. Be playful. Do the things that made you happy and laugh out loud before the cancer. Some responses may have changed, but the feelings they evoked before can still be awakened. Women are sensitive and emotional beings. Intimacy can lead to tears. Let the tears flow to purify the past and step into the new era of what has become and what will be. You are a beautiful soul. Yes, you are a beautiful soul. Let that flow through everything that you are. Feel the true you, then allow your mate to enter your realm of acceptance. You will love more passionately. Love can and will be better after cancer treatment if you allow growth with your significant other. It takes time, but you can do it. Intercourse may be a bit more challenging for some, but there are many ways to make it enjoyable again. Creativity is the key. Why be shy? What do you have to lose? Remember, you thought you were losing your life. Well, now you have a chance to make love to life itself. Enjoy.

Single And/Or Dating After Cancer Treatment

"This is the worst, Doc. I feel so alone. If I could not get anyone before cancer, my chances are really shot now." I stared at her as the tears welled up in her eyes. Inside I prayed, "What can I say to comfort her, Lord?" Silence. I walked over and sat next to her, wiping her tears. I gave her a long hug and just sat there in silence for a while. I heard and I understood. There was truly nothing to say at that point. As our conversation continued, we discussed the body acceptance process, getting involved with hobbies and the community, and doing things that satisfy the soul. The promise of a suitable and accepting mate I could not provide, but that of how to begin living and accepting a new life, I could. We spoke of death and dying and what it means to live from the end, as well as searching for purpose and making a difference. I encouraged her to date and gave her tips on how to later unfold information about the cancer, but only as the relationship would build—no rush. Talking about self-satisfaction made her giggle. Her heart was lifted, and the appointment ended with her more hopeful and with a friendly hug.

<u>Be an Advocate</u>: *Medications can affect libido (desire to have sex) and can also affect your body in other ways (vaginal dryness, stenosis, or narrowing, of the vaginal canal from treatment, and so on). Ask your cancer team if any of the medications or radiation treatment to the pelvis (hip region) will affect future sex and intimacy. Ask for recommendations on how to improve dryness and desires. Remember, you are not the first patient to be treated for this type of cancer, so there is likely to be information that your cancer team can provide.*

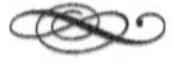

Your happiness lies in you, not in someone else. Continue to enjoy the company of others and be the bold, beautiful person that you are. I will be hopeful with you, that your desires for the right person will bring added happiness. But even if the right person lose their way in finding you, your eternal spring of joy will keep you content and satisfied.

Oh, my dear friend! You're so beautiful! And
your eyes so beautiful—like doves!

—SONG OF SOLOMON 1:15 MSG

Peace, love, and blessings to you—*always*!

CHAPTER 7

Spring: Choosing Life

*Live with intention. Walk to the edge. Listen hard.
Practice wellness. Play with abandon. Laugh. Choose
with no regret. Appreciate your friends. Continue to
learn. Do what you love. Live as if this is all there is.*

—MARY ANNE RADMACHER

NO ONE WAKES UP, HIT the alarm, stretches, and says, "Today, I want to be diagnosed with cancer!" or "Today, I want to have a car accident!" But life happens, and in the end, a choice must be made on how you will adjust to your apprehensions from the chance encounter. Having a car accident may cause someone to never want to drive again or be intimidated by highways. Through counseling, sheer willpower, or the need to drive as part of daily life, some do get behind the wheel again. Others do not but instead choose alternative methods of transportation or rely on family and friends to fulfill their transit needs. Is a cancer diagnosis any different from a car accident experience? Some choose to be like the woman in my dream—dressed, lying in bed, waiting for death. But you can choose the opposite—*life!* After a cancer-diagnosis experience, there is truly no in-between. Should you choose to continue living, you can be certain there will be pauses as well as ups and downs, but keep moving forward steadily with the "new norm" before you. Tears will come, fears will hover, but with the courage of a lioness, inner resolve, and the guidance of the Spirit, you just keep moving forward. Many keep moving forward, because thoughts of "their feet fitting properly in the coffin," like the woman in my dream, are not options on the table.

Cancer recurrence is a cloud that will always be there. Many patients tell me that as the years go by and the tests are less frequent, the cloud gets smaller and smaller. As the fear cloud decreases in size, their hope increases. One lady joked, "With any luck, a quick heart attack will take me out. I'm not into the long, drawn-out business. If anything, the cancer thing allowed me to make peace with others and life." She chuckled as she bid me farewell with a tap on the shoulder and a twinkle in her eyes, the kind of twinkle only seen in the eyes of more mature, wise older women. A knowing. I smiled back, but my heart sighed because I've heard it before and I understood.

CANCER RECURRENCE

Having to tell a patient that they have cancer is the pits, but even worse is having to tell them that the cancer has come back. It seems that patients are now more amenable to being told the reports of scans over the phone—good or bad. I only concur with the latter practice of phone delivery with a few caveats, the most important being that the patient must be home with family and/or friends present or readily available. Having a patient drive in for an appointment to discuss the results of not-so-good news can also be tricky if she must handle heavy machinery, such as driving back home alone. The delivery method is secondary to knowing that the patient has support close by. In today's world of social media, many find themselves very alone. Though they have thousands of friends on the Internet, they have very few trusted friends, if any, in person for support. They don't have a human voice or a human touch. Patients in these situations are the most difficult.

Having practiced for so many years, I have had to deliver the news of cancer recurrence; no physician is ever perfect at it. After reviewing the scan results, I offer support, and if the situation permits, discuss next-step plans. "Can I get more treatments, Doc?" Those hopeful, sad eyes pierce to the heart. Then the silence, deep sighs, and licking and pursing of the lips, as if to inhale and taste life itself. And then comes *the question*: "How much time do I have?" In a majority of cases, this is a tough question for physicians to answer. If the patient is in the intensive care unit (ICU) and kept on medications for life support, we know that if care is withdrawn, then the end is near. Someone walking into my office asking such a question is not the same. I am not a big believer in statistics when the patient is sitting in front of me. The statistics have told us that for the type of cancer, stage, and treatment given, controlling the disease successfully is greater than 80 percent over five years. Yet here the patient is, sitting in my office, one year later, who is now in that 20 percent chance of recurrence. Their odds of recurrence in this patients' case is 100 percent. It's frustrating. But we use the best we have to do the best we know how.

Not all recurrences are immediately life-threatening, though. We have had patients with recurrent metastatic cancer living for many years or even decades with novel treatments. In some cases where treatment is known to be successful after recurrences, I have been able to put the patients' minds at ease by giving better news of possible treatment that can control the disease for years.

A warning of being safe on the highway brings a smile to their faces, even if it is slight. We tend to forget sometimes that common things will be common (a running nose, sneezing is more likely to be allergy than cancer related), and while cancer is fought, there are other simmering health battles, as a patient can still die from other things such as a heart attack—heart disease remains the leading cause of death in this country.

What then? How should the fear of cancer recurrence be handled? I do not have the absolute answer that would suit everyone. What I do have is the truth from patients whom I have been blessed to serve over the years. Cancer recurrences were met with attitudes such as:

* Let's do this. Let's stomp it again!
* If it's my time to go, so be it. Just not too much pain, please.
* I know the time is near. It pains me more than anything to leave my young family behind. But I still want the treatment - the pain…
* I'm not ready to die. I'm going to fight this to the end. Cancer, get ready!
* Life is so beautiful. Shame I'm just seeing it, when I have to go…
* I've been living with this (cancer) recurrence now for five years. I'm tired of being afraid, and I'm afraid of not continuing treatment. I wonder what death is like.
* What are we going to do? Same treatment—again?

As physicians, we cannot say how to respond; we can only offer support and guidance. The answer is within you. There is no expected or standard response. The remainder of the path is yours to take and follow. You must decide how your story will end.

For wisdom is a defense as money is a defense,
But the excellence of knowledge is that
wisdom gives life to those who have it.

—ECCLESIASTES 7:12 NKJV

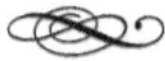

Peace, love, and blessings to you—*always*!

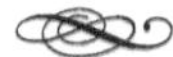

I NEVER THOUGHT I WOULD be writing a book. There are many books available about cancer. Do I really need to add another one? *"Absolutely yes!"* my dear friend countered. "It seems like cancer is much more prevalent than it used to be. Every time I turn around, someone is being diagnosed, or dying from cancer."

She was right. Improved technology over the past few decades have increased our ability to detect cancer at an earlier stage, giving the appearance of *more* cancer being diagnosed. Thanks to the Internet, and conventional and social media coverage, cancer is now less of a tabooed subject. Though valuable information about cancer can be found on the internet, some people may be misguided as well. Many patients report that the information on the internet can be overwhelming and scary. During my guest appearances on radio shows and answering questions at various speaking engagements, it became clear that there are still many unanswered questions about the cancer diagnoses process, treatments options, post-treatment follow-up plans, prevailing myths and so on. Surprisingly, even cancer survivors had questions regarding their past treatments and about how to set up their own survivor care plan, especially when they have received treatments from various locations.

As the request for consultation increased, I noticed much of the initial time was spent addressing common essentials about the cancer journey and how to be an advocate.

Providing copies of my slides and watching audience members take copious notes in various settings, made me realize that there truly appears to be a need. Maybe, there is a role for yet another book. Something simple and short that anyone may use to get the big picture about the cancer journey. One more book just might make a difference.

This book was written because someone just like you felt they need something more. Something simplified. A book that would be *real* and at least mention the apprehension associated with sex and intimacy for women after treatment. I wrote this book from the heart, for you.

This poem was written during the beginning years of my oncology residency training - my eye-opening period, if you will. Every patient diagnosed with cancer has their own story. What do you want out of life? What do you value most?

Thank you for purchasing this book and I hope it was a blessing to you.

With Gratitude,
Your Family Friendly Cancer Doc!
C. M. Williams, M.D.

The Identity of Cancer

I see the patients every day.
I hear the disbelief, the pain, the cry for justification.

4 years old: I'm tired. May I have some chocolate? (My baby should be outside playing—not fair!)

12 years old: What about driving? Can I at least have a learner's permit?

19 years old: I just started college and have plans to do great things.

27 years old: Just finished law school…I've been working so hard for…(sigh).

32 years old: Never have children after treatment? I'm not even dating…(sobs).

40 years old: Not now! I just had a baby—I want to be around…longer.

51years old: What do you mean 50 percent chance of Erectile Dysfunction?

58 years old: I am very angry right now. I have been doing everything right. I am healthy.

63 years old: I am not ready to die yet. I want to see my grandchildren grow up.

78 years old: So many of my friends have gone on…I guess it is my turn now.

86 years old: I had my best golf game in years just last week…no…no.

95 years old: Well, back in my days…what? Hon, I just keep on praying and keep keeping on…

You see…age really does not matter.
Some drew ever closer to God, and others, in defiance, turn away.

And so they came
Rich, poor, middle class,
Blue collar, white collar, orange collar, no collar—living under a bridge
You see, social class does not matter

Please check the box
Eskimo, Black, White non-Hispanic, African American, Native Americans, Hispanic,
Other, none of the above—do not fit in a box?
I am a colorless American
Race, culture, ethnic background is not spared; none is rendered superior.

And so, the ageless, orange-collar, colorless American was diagnosed with cancer
And I watch, in awe, the rebirth and realization of mortality.

C. M. Williams, MD

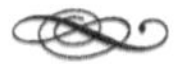

Additional Resources

Since most are visual learners, many have found the video e-Learning website www.Questions4CancerDoctors.com to be very helpful. We also have a booklet, *"Questions for Cancer Doctors – Starter Questions to Encourage Conversations with your Cancer Team."* This booklet will allow patients and caregivers to have an easier time in preparing for appointments and encourages interactive conversations with oncologists. It contains simple questions and area to write down pertinent responses and information. Other established organizations (National Cancer Institute, American Cancer Society, etc.,) can provide verified reading materials on specific cancer, among other resources.

THESE ARE EXAMPLES OF SOME of the commonly known cancers. This list is not complete or exhaustive in any way. Many of the cancer subcategories can be further broken down into tissue types, receptor status, and so on.

Main cancer category	Subcategories of different types of cancers
Breast	Ductal Carcinoma In-situ (DCIS) Invasive disease (infiltrative ductal, lobular carcinoma) Advanced disease
Central Nervous System (CNS); this means the brain and spinal cord	Malignant gliomas Low-grade gliomas Brainstem glioma CNS Lymphoma Ependymomas Meningioma Acoustic neuroma Pituitary tumors Medulloblastoma

The digestive system	Esophageal cancer (swallowing tube) Gastric (stomach) cancer Pancreatic cancer Hepatobiliary cancer -Liver (hepatocellular) -Gallbladder, Bile duct Colon and rectal cancer (Colorectal) Anal cancer
Genitourinary sites	Renal cell carcinoma (kidney) Bladder cancer (male cancers: cancer of penis, prostate cancer, and testicular cancer)
Gynecologic sites	Cervical cancer Endometrial cancer Ovarian cancer Vaginal cancer
Head and neck cancers	Nasopharyngeal cancer (behind nose area) Oropharyngeal cancer (back of mouth) Oral cavity (inside mouth, such as tongue), lip cancers Larynx and hypopharynx cancer (vocal cord area) Salivary gland tumors Thyroid cancers (in front of the neck/Adam's apple area)
Lymphomas and Myeloma	Hodgkin's lymphoma Non-Hodgkin's lymphoma Cutaneous (skin) lymphoma Multiple Myeloma and Plasmacytoma

Musculoskeletal sites	Bone tumors Soft tissue sarcoma
Pediatric (Non-CNS)	Wilms' tumor Neuroblastoma Rhabdomyosarcoma Ewing's sarcoma Pediatric Hodgkin's lymphoma Retinoblastoma
Skin	Basal cell carcinoma (BCC) Squamous cell carcinoma (SCC) Merkel cell carcinoma (MCC) Melanoma/malignant melanoma
Thorax	Small cell lung cancer (SCLC) Non-small-cell lung cancer (NSCLC) Mesothelioma

APPENDIX B
QUESTIONS FOR YOUR CANCER
DOCTORS AND TEAMS

REGARDLESS OF THE EXPERTISE OF the physician you are seeing during a cancer journey, it is always best to have an understanding, no matter how basic, of the upcoming processes. Many patients are embarrassed to ask questions, while others are just unsure of what to ask and therefore just nod their heads, afraid of appearing silly. There is no such thing as a silly or stupid question when your life is on the line. Engage and ask questions until you're satisfied. Your final question should always be, "Is there anything that I should know to be of concern that I am not asking about?"

	Questions to ask
General questions	• Where exactly is the cancer located? Can you show me on an anatomy diagram? (picture of the body?) • Did the cancer spread from where it originated? If yes, where? • What treatment choices do I have? • What treatment do you recommend and why?

Surgeon (local treatment)	• Can you explain clearly and simply, using anatomy pictures of the body, the surgical procedure? • Are there other types of surgery to consider for this cancer? • How long will I be in the hospital after surgery? • What are some of the side effects I can expect once I go home?
Medical oncologist (systemic)	• How will the chemotherapy be given: in pill form or through my vein? • When the chemotherapy makes me sick, what can I take that will make me feel better? • Will I be at risk for sudden bleeding or infection? • After my last dose of chemotherapy, how long can I expect to still have symptoms?
Radiation oncologist (local treatment)	• Can you show me on a diagram where you are going to treat? • Can you show me the organs close by the area being treated and how they may be affected by the radiation? • Are there any special techniques that can be used to protect some of these organs? • Should I be concerned about the risk of getting a second cancer from this treatment?

* For additional simple *visual* cancer e-Learning, visit the ***patient education video website*** at www.Questions4 CancerDoctors.com. Please use "CancerAdvocacy" for a 10 percent discount on their packages.
* Additional questions for appointment can be found in the booklet – *"Questions for Cancer Doctors – Starter Questions to Encourage Conversations with your Cancer Team"*

APPENDIX C
MULTIDISCIPLINARY CLINICS
AND TUMOR BOARDS

A CANCER CLINIC AND/OR TUMOR board discussion is recommended for patients diagnosed with any cancer. A clinic is frequently done for more common cancers, such as breast and prostate, but at a minimum, a tumor board is recommended, as noted in the definition within the book. This list is not complete, but should only be used as a guide to give an idea of what can be expected and to engage in conversation with your physician about *who actually is and who should be on your team.*

Specialty	What they do for you
Surgery (local treatment)	The goal of surgery is to safely remove the bulk of the cancer. Some areas may be more challenging than others. Other treatments may be given first to try and decrease the size the of the cancer prior to attempting surgery

51

Medical oncology (systemic)	**Chemotherapy:** This treatment goes all over the body and is therefore considered "systemic," meaning it goes everywhere (if anywhere on the body is cut and bleeding, then chemotherapy can go to that location). The drug seeks to destroy any microscopic cancer cells (those that cannot be seen by the naked eye) that may have gotten into the vascular system (blood and lymphatics). Normal tissues/cells are destroyed in the process, but normal cells repair themselves (such as hair regrowth), while the cancer cells cannot repair themselves and are destroyed. **Targeted Therapies:** All cells have antennae that serve different functions. Cancer cells also have antennae that may be signaling the cancer cells to grow, or they affect other functions, not allowing the cancer cells to be turned off and/or die when they should. Targeted therapies serve to block these antennae, and their ultimate goal is destroying the cancer cells.

*Radiation oncology (local treatment)	**External:** Just like getting an x-ray, nothing will be felt during the actual treatment, where powerful x-rays are used to treat the area that the cancer is located. Additively, you will experience side effects similar to getting a progressive sunburn (the effects on the breast, the rectum, and lung will all be different). Your doctor will explain more based on cancer location. **Internal:** This requires a procedure that places a "radioactive source" (think of it as a small pebble that gives off radiation) close to the affected area, which is then exposed for a few minutes before the source is removed. Practical example: sun-tanning for a short period of time.
Pathology	This looks at the biopsied tissue sample under a microscope that enlarges the cells. This allows differentiation of normal cells from cancer cells. Many stains are also done to provide additional information to guide treatment (example: Estrogen Receptors (ER) in breast cancer)

*Radiologists	Different types of imaging allow us to see inside the body that may show us things that are abnormal and/or does not belong in certain areas. More than one imaging type may be required to further clarify what is being seen. Examples: Mammogram may show something that requires an Ultrasound to see it better. A Brain CT scan may require an MRI to further characterize an abnormality. After a CT scan of the chest, abdomen and pelvis a PET scan, may be required to find out if a mass is active with cancer or not.
Genetics	A cancer diagnosis to a younger-age patient or one with a certain type of cancer may prompt your team to ask you to consider genetic testing. Be sure to have a discussion as to what is being looked for and how the information will add to the treatment process. (For example: a forty-eight-year-old woman with right breast cancer whose mother and aunt had breast and ovarian cancer may consider a genetic panel. The results would help with the decision regarding lumpectomy versus mastectomies, future cancer risk reduction, and how to educate her daughters regarding their future cancer risks.)

Rehabilitation	After any surgical procedure, a period of readjustment is required. Depending on the type of cancer, rehabilitation can sometimes be extensive. This can include various services that focus on different aspects of the body. (For example: cancer of the head and neck requires speech and swallowing evaluation and rehabilitation after surgery, dental services before and after surgery, and so on. Others include, but are not limited to, physical therapy, occupational therapy, and speech therapy.) These clinics assist with making the activities of daily living more manageable.
Psychosocial	Cancer diagnosis is difficult to handle by yourself, no matter your inner reserve and strength. A discussion of the cancer encounter and how it affects your home, work, and social life will help with establishing that "new normal" we previously discussed. Be honest, open, and candid with yourself. It tends to help you make a more transparent assessment of where you are and not where you think you should be. Remember, there are no set expected or standard responses to a cancer diagnosis.

Clinical trials	The treatment recommendations we have today are based on past trials and studies that other patients thankfully participated in. Clinical trials seek to answer questions on ways to improve treatment, decrease toxicity (side effects), and have the same or better outcomes. Before embarking on a clinical trial, be sure to understand how it is formatted, the clinical questions the study seek to answer, expected side effects, the possibility of getting the real treatment versus no treatment (placebo), and so on. Even if you decided not to participate, it is good to consider and review information and make an informed decision.
Nutrition	This is important before, during, and after cancer treatment. Some treatments may affect your ability to eat, digest, or taste food. Maintaining an ideal weight and good nutrition is vital. Engage your nutritionist to teach you more.

*Be sure to understand the difference between a radiation oncologist and a radiologist. In a hospital setting, you may be sent to the wrong department if it is unclear what service you seek, which can be very frustrating.

A ***radiation oncologist*** uses radiation to treat cancer (not radiology oncology—the mention of *radiology* causes routing to the radiology section as many are not familiar with the word "oncology"). ***Radiologists*** review the imaging required to diagnose a variety of ailments (not just cancer)—CT scan, chest x-ray, MRI, mammogram, and so on.

Claustrophobic? If you need an MRI, be sure to let the ordering physician know *before* the scan. He or she can prescribe something for you to relax.

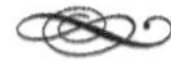

www.ingramcontent.com/pod-product-compliance
Lightning Source LLC
Chambersburg PA
CBHW031422250726
48656CB00002B/789